How To Satisfy Her Simply: Simple tips to give your woman multiple satisfaction sexually

James E. Mayer

Table of Contents

Chapter 1
Chapter 2
Chapter 3

Chapter 1

Setting up a sexy environment

With regards to getting a charge out of sex in the room, it's less about the style and more about the little components that make a room more exotic but, pleasurably agreeable.
If you've been together for some time, room sex can wind up turning out to be very exhausting and unsurprising sooner or later. You realize the specific way the cushion feels. The natural snorts and groans. Also, there's nothing new to wrinkle things up. Also, very much like all the other things throughout everyday life, if you truly need to keep the fervor and the expectation alive, you want to make new encounters in the room constantly.

For what reason do we have to keep the enthusiasm alive?

Before we discuss the most ideal ways to transform your drilling room into a provocative room, there's another thing you want to recollect. What's more, that is keeping the energy and fervor alive in a relationship.

The initial not many weeks or months of another relationship are generally novel and invigorating. What's more, the main justification for why it's so flank-shivering and energizing is the result of the capriciousness in the relationship. Both of you are as yet finding out about other, and each and everything both of you do together is an exceptional encounter.

As the relationship develops and you've invested sufficient energy in one another's arms, the shiver begins to blur. Yet, you need to attempt to reproduce that uniqueness as frequently as you can even as the years cruise by. To guarantee that you make one-of-a-kind sexual recollections, accomplish something that will bring both

of you closer physically, and keep your
sexual coexistence alive.
You could go out for a heartfelt, calm supper
or you could go clubbing and let the force of
a PDA warm both of your flanks up.
Whatever seems best for you is simply great,
since adoration and erotic nature are
however interesting as the couple that you
may be.

At the point when you go out on the town,
you make a previously unheard-of memory.
Furthermore, that generally prompts better
things when you return home, particularly if
both of you are physically stirred around
one another. So however much we center
around the best sex room thoughts to tidy
up your room and transform it into an
underhanded, hot room, you likewise need
to ensure you keep the sentiment alive!
Now that we've zeroed in on the significance
of keeping the energy alive, we should take a
gander at the best sex room thoughts to

make a hot room that overflows with erotic nature each time you're sleeping!

You've heard those weak remarks about the room being "where the wizardry occurs," yet this banality is valid, unfortunately.
The wizardry occurs in the room. It can occur on top of your clothing machine too, however, the room is fundamentally your sex base. In this way, if your hot time is everything except otherworldly, a decent spot to begin is by making a provocative room. Consider this minor remodel utilizing these sex room thoughts as a venture into your sexual into existe

1. Stay away from white
White is spotless and flawless looking, in any case, assuming that you're truly anticipating engaging in sexual relations, don't have white sheets. You would rather not have dull sex. You need to have crude, muddled sex. White won't give you that.

White will have you restless the entire time, ensuring you won't stain the sheets.

More obscure sheets, particularly red ones look antique yet exotic. Then again, red or orange drapes can give your room that sexy shine as well. However at that point once more, be cautious with an excess of red in the room. Get out of hand, and your room might begin to seem to be an exaggerated massage parlor.

2. Lighting is everything
On the off chance that you need a provocative room, lighting is everything, it represents the deciding moment in a room.

On the off chance that you have glaring lights, commit to never turning those frightful things on, and purchase a standing light all things being equal. Your lighting ought to be delicate and faint. If it's too dull, there's insufficient visual excitement. In any case, a lot of light is damaging.

With regards to a hot and heartfelt room, recall that milder, smooth lighting is in every case better to assist you with setting the temperament. At the point when you utilize milder, yellowish lighting that looks like a consuming chimney, you feel hotter and quieter, your skin shines better, and everything simply looks hotter!

Also, the most awesome aspect of this sex room thought is that the delicate light mixes out all that cellulite and muscle-to-fat ratio on your body while you're having intercourse. Also, that will just cause you to have good expectations about your own body, and a spotlight on the better things close by!

3. Get into the surface
Attempt to integrate different surfaces into your room since it'll uplift the faculties. Rather than your fundamental cotton sheets, attempt silk. It'll be somewhat strange from the outset, yet there's

something extremely erotic about it that you'll develop to adore. Feel free to mess about and see what surfaces help you out in the room.

4. Silk robes and attractive undergarments

However much these provocative room tips are tied in with making an exotic environment, the ideal love stylistic layout is deficient without both of you filling the role. Incredible sex is about the sensation, however, you can continuously increase the sensation with engaging clothing. Continuously spruce up for bed, regardless of whether the garments fall off in almost no time. Your bodies resemble wonderful presents, and very much like anything invigorating, it generally looks best assuming it's gift-wrapped flawlessly. Wear elegant underwear or free silk robes that uncover, yet not totally. Entice your accomplice and excite them, yet don't uncover all until you're now in the demonstration.

5. Set up sexy craftsmanship

Presently, you needn't bother with a lot of bare photographs to cause a space to feel hot. Photographs of your family are great, in any case, perhaps keep them out of the room if you have any desire to at any point have energetic sex once more. Family photographs and sex room thoughts simply don't blend quite well!

Your accomplice would rather not be gazing at your mother while they're going to climax. On the off chance that craftsmanship isn't your thing, in any event, draping an image of a scene is not the best, but not terrible either than nothing.

6. Lose the workplace look

Having a monster work area in your room with a lot of wires and papers spread out wherever won't give you a hot room vibe.

Truth be told, it gives a greater amount of office energy, and that dream possibly works assuming you're engaging in sexual relations in an office. It kills the sexual energy that you're attempting to make in your room. Thus, keep your own life separate from work.

7. Delicate sheets

Delicate sheets are wizardry while you're brushing your bum against it, particularly as you move your pelvises as one. Put resources into at least 600 string count Egyptian cotton sheets, and ensure they're spotless *and fragrant as well, on the off chance that you're attempting to be posh*. At the point when you engage in sexual relations, each sensation is featured, and a great many people overlook sheets. Try not to be that individual, since great sheets truly have an effect!

8. The right bedding

Your accomplice ought to awaken in your bed feeling beyond, dislike they've been hit by a transport. Put in a couple of additional dollars and help yourself out by getting a steady and agreeable bed. Well, you'll be the one dozing in it the most, so it's true to your greatest advantage.

There are two things to recollect here. Solid bedding gives you great help while resting. Furthermore, a delicate sleeping pad clincher could your body at any point sink in as you lie on top of your accomplice, giving you both a cozy inclination, and a more profound entrance. So settle on what you need, and get something that feels great, and hot!

9. An agreeable floor

It's insane exactly the number of horny rabbits that wind up having awkward sex or experiencing excruciating rug consumes and knees scratches since they chose to have intercourse on the floor to keep things somewhat more unusual and energizing!

If you're wanting to make out anyplace past the bed, put resources into a thick and delicate floor covering. Keep in mind, the delight of sex is in the synchrony of two bodies, however, the base you're lying on has a major impact on keeping the energy alive. Having intercourse on a terrible base resembles engaging in sexual relations near the ocean. Everybody "thinks" it's hot until you attempt it and understand it's dreadful by any means. And afterward, you have sand inside your vagina for the entire following week!

Lay a thick, delicate carpet, in some piece of the room, so you have more space to get imaginative and evaluate other extravagant situations on the floor.

10. Slender, sheer sheets

How can anybody manage sheer sheets lying around a room? Indeed, you can utilize it to increase the joy of sex!

You can utilize delicate, sheer sheets to outline your accomplice and joy them up from over the sheets or blindfold them with silk scarves or by utilizing a delicate cushion. Utilize the faculties to energize your accomplice, enacting each sense in turn. It'll stir your accomplice significantly more than energizing every one of the five faculties without a moment's delay.

11. Sex furniture

If you can bear the cost of this extra, sex furniture simply makes a sex room much more tomfoolery and mischievous! A chaise parlor would work impeccably as well if you have the space for it. Oron the other hand, you could go with a wedge on the bed, that works as well!

12. Get a few candles rolling

Whether you're a man or a lady, everybody likes candles. It adds a heartfelt touch to your provocative room, it resembles tying a bow on a gift.

If certain about something, however, don't get scented candles except if you understand what you're doing. Certain individuals don't respond excessively well to them, and a portion of those candles smell like blossomed upchuck. Along these lines, if all else fails, go unscented.

13. Mirrors

Mirrors are hot, they're truly hot. Have you at any point seen yourself having intercourse in a mirror? Do it. Something doesn't add up about it that only amps up the sexual energy.

Presently, you don't need to tile your entire roof in mirrors. In any case, having a standing mirror in the corner adds that wrinkle to the hot room.

14. Keep a clean room

Individuals like clean individuals. Indeed, that is a stunning disclosure! Keep your room clean. It doesn't need to be flawless, you're just human. In any case, if any messy garments are on the floor, just put them in the pantry. Vacuum frequently. You know, essential cleanliness. A hot room is a spotless one.

15. Aphrodisiacs

Your sex room is most certainly inadequate without these little consumable love enhancers. It doesn't make any difference if it's chocolate syrup, consumable body paint, or seasoned lubes, as long as you give something to bed to upgrade the joy.

The room is one of the most widely recognized at this point exhausting spots to have intercourse. In any case, if you can transform that repetitive room sex into something energizing and tomfoolery utilizing these sex room thoughts, something that endures longer and feels more pleasurable, why not use it and bring the flashback?

16. Ensure you dispose of interruptions

If you have a television in your room, dispose of it, or use it just to play some pornography while you're engaging in sexual relations. A provocative room is a spot for two things: having intercourse and resting. Furthermore, ensure you have a spot to put your wireless so you will not be occupied on the off chance that you get an instant message or call.

17. Mind-set music

Once in a while, quiet can be a major interruption in bed. You can discuss your dreams or groan going to mute the quiet, yet nothing beats music in bed to bring the mood back into the pelvic pushing!

Music goes about as a guide in deciding the sexual energy that will happen. The right sort of music can cause you to have harsh sex, energetic sex, or even sluggish sex - And everything relies upon the energy you both feel with the music. Keep a couple of hot playlists prepared consistently, so you don't need to go searching for a decent one. On the off chance that you needed to pick one to circle endlessly, pick one from this untouched best rundown of the hot lovemaking playlist.

18. Scents and oils

A provocative room is never finished without scents and oils. Presently, slathering oil on one another may not be something you can do each evening, what with every one of the slick sheets the following morning. Yet, this can be a periodic extravagance that can be enjoyed.

Foreplay is somewhat significant for drawn-out sex, and ladies love a man who can enjoy long foreplay. Yet, if one of you loves gathering the speed up, scented body oils are an extraordinary method for dragging out the demonstration of sex. Rather than skipping foreplay, run the oil over your accomplice as they lounge in the warm shine of glimmering candles. It's energetic, and hot and feels so tricky and wet when you're on top of one another.

For most different evenings, lighting a sexy incense or simply utilizing a regular diffuser with rejuvenating balms would work similarly as well!

19. Toss a few cushions on the bed
Pads shout solace in a hot room. Assuming you just have two pads, your bed looks miserable. Add a couple of cushioned pads since it gives more non-abrasiveness and solace to your space. Likewise, those cushions will prove to be useful to put under

somebody's butt for a lift, or in any event, when you snuggle a while later.

20. Try not to have a nursery in your room

You most likely heard that plants make your place homier, in any case, not in your room. You can have a plant or two, however, don't go over the top. Additionally, on the off chance that you realize you will not have the option to deal with them, then quit this. Nobody needs to engage in sexual relations close to something kicking the bucket.

21. Adopt a more grown-up strategy

Assuming you were a top-pick football player in secondary school, that is perfect. In any case, we don't have to see every decoration you at any point won holding tight to your wall. You need to move into your life and go with a more grown-up look. Your achievements are something to be glad

for, however, don't make your room seem to
be the Lobby of Notoriety.

22. Put your character in it

If you utilize these sex room thoughts we've
shared up until this point, you're ensured to
have a room that slimes sex bid. Yet, you
need to ensure that your character shows in
your room. Pick things that you like and that
you believe are hot, because then, at that
point, it will make it a one-of-a-kind spot to
communicate and encounter your form of
sexual energy.

We should not burn through any additional
time. With these sex room thoughts and
little fixes, you can change your drilling
room into a hot room in a day. So why not
get everything rolling, and set up your bed
for brilliant sex and wild times?!

Chapter 2

The indispensable foreplay tactics

.Foreplay is something we will generally disregard on occasion yet is a fundamental piece of intercourse. For ladies, it allows them to 'heat' up and get in that frame of mind. It likewise permits them to now and again arrive at the climax. Numerous men are ignorant however the normal sound male endures roughly 5 minutes before arriving at peak while the typical solid female can require as much as 17 minutes to arrive at the peak. This is known as the climax hole.

Did you know an investigation of more than 8,000 ladies showed that just 6% of ladies arrive at climax through penile-vaginal intercourse? (Kontula, Miettinen, 2016) Along these lines, on the off chance that your skip foreplay chances are that she isn't getting a charge out of sex as much as you.

Also, on the off chance that you think she will be, she's most probably faking it.

Before we hop into the great stuff, we should discuss the female life structures.
The Female Life systems and Why Foreplay Is Significant
The female body is more convoluted than the male's body. She's not normally prepared to get going on orders.
Match that with the way that ladies are more invigorated by contact than sight, and you have all the comprehension you want about why foreplay for ladies is significant.

What Is The Clitoris?
The clitoris is the main issue of joy in a lady's body.
While there are nerves all through the vulva and inside the vagina, this is where the joy place is arranged.

Where Could The Clitoris be?

The clitoris is simpler to find than most folks anticipate. The inward labia (lips) structure a hood right over the clitoris, which is a little bud that somewhat projects outward. The clitoral hood safeguards the clitoris from direct feeling. With somewhere around 15,000 sensitive spots gathered into one region, direct contact can be naturally extraordinary.

What Is The Sweet Spot?

What and Where is the Female Sweet Spot In 1950, a German gynecologist by the name of Ernst Gräfenberg found a spot inside the vagina that, when animated, created massive sexual joy. In some cases, the excitement of the spot can make a lady discharge.

The fortunate person named the spot after himself: the Gräfenberg spot, which has for quite some time been abbreviated to simply Sweet spot (fortunately!).

Where Is The Sweet Spot?
Finding the Sweet spot is somewhat more earnest than tracking down the clitoris. This marginally raised, somewhat rough spot lies in the internal upper mass of the vagina, and only one out of every odd female can pinpoint precisely where the spot is found, however, experimentation is loads of fun during foreplay.

The Main 19 Foreplay Tips And Thoughts For Men

1. Prepare The Space For Sex
Romantic Setting Ladies Love
A ton of folks have this limited focus capacity to focus on the thing they're doing and fail to remember all the other things during sex. Ladies will more often than not get
diverted effectively by their current circumstance and that rundown of things that should be finished.

Assuming that you welcome her in the room, get some margin to clear the messiness, fix the sheets, get your clothing, and for the most part clean up the living space.

It never damages to set the stage all things considered. Faint the lights, light a candle, turn on some music, or possibly, switch off YouTube.

2. Take as much time as is needed Stripping down

Ways Of Turning Her On Before Sex
Assuming you're going for foreplay ladies like, remember that it is undeniably more enticing and exciting if you require some investment stripping away the layers of attire. Indeed, it tends to be difficult to take on a steady speed when you need to get your eyes all around her body.

She will see the value in the expectation that shows up with eliminating each piece of clothing in turn and the consideration you give her body all the while.

Take off her shirt and stroke her shoulders and arms. Pull off her jeans, gradually, and kiss or contact her legs and thighs as you do. Eliminate her bra and touch her bosoms. Pull off her undies and ... you understand.

3. Make The Clitoris And Sweet Spot On the way Places, Not Your Beginning stages

Didn't your mom show you not to have dessert before supper?
The clitoris and Sweet spot are significant focuses to being aware of a lady's body, however, foreplay ought to never begin here. Foreplay before sex is tied in with empowering her to prepare heated up and.

Making a plunge directly into clitoral feeling or Sweet spot excitement doesn't work if she's not undoubtedly somewhat stirred as of now.

4. Dial It Back, Form Expectation

Pump the brakes in The Room

Getting somewhat more top to bottom with tip three above, dialing back is something that can make all the difference for your foreplay endeavors, and it is one of the foreplay tips for men that can be the greatest battle.

Indeed, you are energized, as is she, however, you need to develop something unimaginably critical to the, generally speaking, sexual experience: expectant delight. Easing back your role is the least complex method for doing that.

The human mind knows two essential types of delight:

Expectant - Joy experienced fully expecting something we need. Consider the inclination you get when you truly need that pizza and the conveyance driver shows up.
Consummatory - Joy experienced when you get what you've been needing. That euphoria you feel when you dive into the main chomp of pizza.

With regards to sex, developing sexual pressure and accomplishing uplifted conditions of joy is about expectation, and expectation falls right at the focal point of sexual delight.
Additionally, it works something very similar for the two guys and females.

A few people struggle with dialing back, particularly on the off chance that foreplay is a two-way road and she's contributed a ton of excitement to you.
This is where a desensitizing splash like Promescent can truly be a redeeming quality. Particularly assuming that you expect to perform ineffectively in bed.

5. Go ahead and Seek clarification on some things

Couple Seeking clarification on pressing issues and Imparting
You want to stimulate her, yet if you're battling with nailing down what she loves, simply inquire. Joost ladies value direct

inquiries; it shows her that you plan to satisfy her how she gets a kick out of the chance to be satisfied, and that can be a turn-on without help from anyone else.

Try not to allow your inquiries to be adolescent. Put some thought into them, or utilize the way that you want direction as a valuable chance to infuse some filthy talk.

For instance:
Show me where you need my hands.
Do you like it when I rub your (embed hot body part name) like this?
Let me know how you believe that I should manage my mouth.
Regardless of whether your accomplice is a bit modest in the room, the course of her appearance you things she enjoys without having to straightforwardly answer can be unimaginably hot for both of you. Also, you get the direction you're looking for in foreplay thoughts. It's a shared benefit one way or the other.

6. Escape The Room ... Or on the other hand The House

Lady Unsatisfied in The Room

Sex doesn't need to happen just in the room, and foreplay doesn't by the same token. A great deal of energy can show up by evaluating some erotic play in different rooms in the house.

Start foreplay in the lounge, while she's collapsing clothing, or slip into the shower with her and kick the party off. Regardless of whether you end up in the room, in the end, messing about in new spots and circumstances can truly get her warmed up and energized.

Remember that escaping the house can truly raise sexual encounters higher than ever. Lease a lodging for the night a couple of towns away and go on a street outing for certain distinctly arranged stops en route for some biased foreplay.

7. Get Spotless, Get Prepped, And Get Attractive

Man With Great Cleanliness
Do you know how you are captivated by clean skin and a well-manicured shock under provocative underwear? In all honesty, this is similarly as tempting for ladies. NOT the provocative undies — except if that she's into, then ... let it all out. Being perfect, smelling pleasant, and slipping into a decent set of hot clothing is one of the simplest ways of exciting a lady.

Do a little manscaping.
She'll see the value in the endeavors regardless of whether she expresses it without holding back.

8. Permit Her To Start leading the pack When She Needs To

If you're the person who generally prefers to be in control in the room, it tends to be somewhat obnoxious assuming your accomplice starts to lead the pack, however, it is very worth the effort to let her.

Show her you like it when she's the initiator by answering and empowering her to start to lead the pack. You wouldn't believe how turned on she gets when she is coordinating every one of the moves.

9. Kiss Her, Yet Kiss Her Right

Exotic foreplay is about enthusiastic touch that may not include genitalia by any means, and kissing is one of the most seasoned types of erotic foreplay for ladies.

How you kiss says a lot to a lady. If you've figured out how to get drool all around her face, you're doing everything wrong.

Assuming you understand what her tonsils taste like, she's presumably going to feel abused.

If you've dried out her lips from a lot of pecking, it's a misstep.

Kiss her delicately however immovably, and don't simply zero in on her mouth. Allow your kisses to wander to her neck, ears, and cheeks.

Also, don't keep your lips stuck on her the whole time. Simply blend the kisses in.

10. Keep in mind, Foreplay Starts Outside The Room

Foreplay begins far before you at any point contact her.

If you've ignored her for the greater part of the day, been excessively occupied to offer her much consideration, or are generally oblivious to her necessities past the room, it will be more diligently to get her in that frame of mind, regardless of how great the genuine foreplay is.

Set aside some margin to tell her she's critical to you, that she's at the forefront of your thoughts, and that you need her well before you at any point attempt to infuse foreplay to prepare her for sex

11. Think of Her as A [Dirty] Love Letter

Compose a Heartfelt Letter

Love letters have sort of kicked the bucket
with the introduction of electronic
correspondence, yet a written-by-hand letter
is a lot more significant.

A letter conveying your adoration is perfect,
however, zest it up a little. Tell her how you
like it when she does specific things during
or before sex.

Let her know it's about her body that gets
your blood streaming.

Advise her on how you need to treat her.

12. Utilize Your Enchanted Fingers For An Exotic Backrub

Sex and sexual contact are perfect, however
erotic back rub is another universe of joy for
her. The erotic back rub will cause her to
feel like she's supported, revered, and
cherished, and getting her casual aides bring
down her hindrances from there on.

Thus, for an exceptional treat, bring down
the lights, tenderly take off her dress and

give her a sluggish and provocative rubdown.

13. Talk A Bit, However, Don't Go on and on

Being a tease Ladies The Correct Way
A little messy talk is a pleasant method for warming things up yet proceed cautiously with those words you use to get your woman in that frame of mind and calibrate your grimy conversing with her inclinations. Each lady is unique — however much that makes your work harder as the person who's meaning to satisfy her. A few women will be irritated with one too many shoptalk terms for her woman parts.

A few ladies like it if you accomplish such a great deal of messy talking that the crudest mariner would become flushed. A few ladies are most stirred by heartfelt words and cherishing phrases during foreplay.

Hello, it takes various types, so sort out what your accomplice likes and express out loud whatever she jumps at the chance to hear.

Something else to remember: Avoid that flinch-initiating, antique expressions. (You know the ones — think low-spending plan pornography.)

14. Discuss Your Sexual Dreams Including Her

All kinds of people appreciate realizing that their accomplice fantasizes about them doing specific things. Regardless of whether she's not sharing her dreams right now, inform her concerning your own, regardless of whether you are somewhat timid and need to get them on paper.

She may simply step up and satisfy your dreams, and, surprisingly better, she might unveil to you her very own portion.

This personal trade of fantastical thoughts can get things warmed up quicker than you can envision — on the two finishes.

15. Construct A Foreplay Tool compartment
Promescent Foreplay Tool stash.
A couple of clever instruments can truly perk up foreplay before sex. You don't need to go hard and fast, yet fix up a foreplay tool stash you can go after on the end table or under the bed.
A decent, essential foreplay unit ought to include:

A decent water-based lube or a characteristic lube like coconut oil
A fundamental vibrator for her (a little wand or vibrating egg works pleasant)
A couple of lightweight servitude toys for good measure, as delicate wrist limitations or a blindfold
The foreplay tool stash can be essentially as comprehensive as you like it to be, however

having the fundamentals close by shows you're good to go.

16. Properly investigate things
Do Exploration on Foreplay Methods
Google is your dearest companion for finding foreplay tips for men.
A lot of men battle about knowing different foreplay strategies.
In any case, there's no disgrace in involving Google or your #1 web crawler and composing in something like foreplay thoughts or how to foreplay for instance.

You can glean tons of useful knowledge by perusing different illustrative aids like this, recordings about foreplay, and pictures that exhibit charts.
Another extraordinary asset is schoolofsquirt.com

All ladies are unique and there are different things you ought to find out about knowing how the female body functions. It simply requires a little investment and exertion however you will be happy you did thus will she.

17. Give Her A greater amount of What She Needs

Giving Her A greater amount of What She Needs

On the off chance that you've been with your accomplice for some time, you presumably have a smart thought of what she loves in the foreplay division, and nothing bad can be said about doing what you know works, regardless of whether it appears to be standard.

If she answers well to a sexy back rub, give it to her. Assuming that she cherishes oral sex, oblige her, joyfully. If she loves a specific toy, use it.

It's fine to investigate and attempt new things, yet the believed foreplay that has consistently worked ought to never be

placed as a second thought since you need to
have a go at a novel, new thing.

18. Mess With just the right amount of BDSM.

You may not think you (or she) would be all
that inspired by BDSM during foreplay,
however unusual BDSM doesn't need to
mean calfskin outfits and whips.
Certain individuals are shocked at exactly
how much excitement can show up with a
bit:

- Beating
- Light gnawing
- Controlling

Give it a shot with your accomplice, and
welcome her to concoct a protected word
you both can utilize if both of you feel
awkward.

19. Realize When To Forego The Foreplay And Only Put it all on the line

Indeed, foreplay is significant, magnificent, whatnot and whatnot, hips for your sexual coexistence.

Be that as it may, now and again, skirting the foreplay and going ideal for the gold is entirely fine. The key here is you need to get to realize your accomplice alright to know when she's all prepared for the taking without the commonplace support.

In some cases, if you two are holding a sexual meaning to your relationship, the broiler will as of now be preheated without you having to press any buttons physically. In this way, it'll be entirely fine to get cooking.

Conclusion

Foreplay for ladies gets her turned on before you go any further.

Not at all like men, ladies aren't normally prepared for sex when it gets everything

rolling; their actual excitement process is much more muddled.
As a little something extra, great foreplay time for her draws her nearer to the objective of peaking, and that implies you'll be less inclined to complete first before she's done whenever sex is started.

Utilizing a defer splash as Promescent will likewise be of mense in that area.

Chapter 3

The 'inside-out' tactics

Penis Pushing Tips to Give Your Lady an Extraordinary Encounter

In all honesty, there is a workmanship to entering your lady and how you push all through her pussy. It's not all pretty much drilling away as you found in pornography. Certainly, she might like it rigid at certain focuses during sex, yet odds are good that she will appreciate it more assuming that you fluctuate your pushes a little.

The principal thing to comprehend is that ladies love the primary push. Every lady I've at any point been with will let out a major groan when she feels you enter her completely interestingly.
Realizing this I generally prefer to prod a little and develop some expectations before sliding in completely the initial time. This

typically includes scouring your penis head on the all-around of her pussy lips and scouring the tip of your penis on her clitoris. Something else I like to do is slide my penis all over the beyond her vagina, but not enter her. Consider a frank sliding all through a bun. Also, you can constantly rest the tip of your penis at the kickoff of her vagina while you kiss, and so forth. (This will drive her wild.)

There are two fundamental sorts of pushing.

The shallow push and the profound push. Shallow pushing permits you to invigorate the launch of her vagina up to about an inch down, which for some ladies is an exceptionally delicate piece of the vagina. Likewise, the launch of her vagina is in many cases the most impenetrable part, so shallow pushes permit you to focus a lot of excitement on the top of your penis and just underneath, which feels wonderful.

The profound push can be incredibly pleasurable for both of you. There's nothing very like the sensation of being completely inside your lady and hearing her groan with delight. Profound pushing can permit you to go for the gold spot and it can likewise permit you to situate your pelvic bone on her clitoris or the region around her clitoris permitting her to rub facing you to set off a clitoral climax. I make sense of a method called the Feline here that turns out perfect for giving her a clitoral climax during the entrance.

One thing to note about profound pushing is that assuming your lady's vagina is especially shallow or your penis is especially lengthy, diving too deep too quick, so remember that could be awkward.

Eventually, you'll need to explore different avenues regarding both profound and shallow pushes with fluctuating paces. Not exclusively will changing your pushing style give her a mind-boggling experience, yet it can likewise assist you with enduring longer during sex. For instance, one of my number one maneuvers is to give my lady five or so profound pushes and afterward, on the 6th one, push profound and simply leave my penis somewhere within her vagina for about a second or something like that, and assuming your lady is doing Kegel works out, she can press your penis with her vagina simultaneously. Accept me this feels astonishing and permits you to ensure you don't overwhelm yourself excessively fast. If you want to realize every one of my methods for enduring longer during sex, look at my Outrageous Endurance course here.

Like with any sexual method, the key is to keep an open line of correspondence with your accomplice and attempt bunches of various pushing styles, and right away you'll find what drives her wild and gives you extreme joy.

This one strategy is answerable for in a real sense a huge number of climaxes from ladies everywhere. While it's really easy to pull off it's likewise Extremely strong. Try not to be astonished assuming she even spurts from it, truth be told.

I exhibit the procedure on record in a tasteful, clean way utilizing a daily existence like a model of the vagina so you will know precisely how to make it happen.

Men can have somewhat of a drill way to deal with pushing, loads of strain, and snugness, which can be alright on the off chance that you're zeroing in on contact to acquire excitement as opposed to feeling. To move into more profound, more associated love production you'll have to dominate a more extensive collection of pushes. However, it's not only the men. Intercourse isn't just a man pushing into an uninvolved accomplice. She should be participated in her pelvis and move with the movement as well. Preferably you're moving in a symphonious harmony. So these focuses, while coordinated to men, apply to the lady as well. (Furthermore, statements of regret for being so heterocentric, it applies at whatever point a penis or phallic item is moving all through an accomplice.)

Significant Point #1: Loosen up your hips

Keep your pelvic region loose, hips, bum, and tummy. You'll feel more, you'll have more command over your developments, you'll be more delicate about how your accomplice's body is answering, and you'll move all the more openly and easily.

Significant Point #2: Spotlight on the Out as much as the In

As opposed to zeroing in on the in-in, which gives a jerky extraordinary feel to the push, center around the out as much as the in.

This gives a more sexy streaming feel to the push.

It likewise implies that as opposed to your accomplice preparing herself against the consistent flood of pushes, she also gets into a streaming musicality of inviting in the push, drawing in with it, and afterward delivering with the outward development. It keeps a dynamic of needing and getting going that keeps up with high conditions of excitement for extensive periods.

Significant Point #3: Shift the Beat

Consider your pushing like music - you don't maintain that it should be steady extreme whip metal! Nor do you maintain that it should be a steady lead-up to a fabulous crescendo. Like great music, a decent meeting of adoration causes will be chan, times of force sprinkled with gentler developments.

Significant Point #4: Change the Stroke

It's not all profound pushing in and out. In some cases, you'll just push shallowly with the top of your penis at the passage of her vagina. Some of the time you'll be as far as possible in and push shallowly, just moving a bit. Some of the time you'll scatter shallow pushes with profound pushes - attempt a cadence of five shallow to one profound. Some of the time you'll push gradually step by step, further and more profoundly. Some of the time you should push more to the sides than straight in, or you could attempt circles or all the more a crushing impact.

Significant Point #5: Bang with your Body, not your Penis

To give the feeling of banging hard, which can feel better for the lady if she's in the temperament for it, as opposed to jabbing hard with your penis, swing in with your hips with your body weight behind it. At the point when gotten along admirably (and check in with her to know this) this will give a flood of delight all through her body.

Significant Point #5: Deal with Your Excitement

At the point when you become amazing at the push you can keep going for a long time. The casual swing of the push permits you to deal with your excitement levels, keeping you at an elevated state without spilling into discharge. If you feel yourself getting excessively near the edge, change the idea of the push, dialing back, moving less, stopping, or evolving position.

Pushing in this manner feels perfect for a lady and gives her the fundamental excitement to have the option to go into elevated conditions of excitement herself, having rushes of climaxes that flood her entire body.

It's workmanship worth dominating!

5 Sex Places That Will Make Any Lady Groan

What about climaxes is, that they are subtle and some of the time, you simply need to counterfeit them. Presently you've made it happen so frequently thus well, you're in line for an Oscar. Have you at any point contemplated whether it's simply you? No, honey. Allow me to break it to you, most ladies find it challenging to climax during standard intercourse. No, Do-It-Yourself isn't the arrangement. Assume responsibility for your climaxes and request what is legitimately yours.

Presently here's a central issue. Any lady who says she can climax just by sex is lying! Furthermore, on the off chance that she's not, poach her man. Clitoris excitement and foreplay are fundamental. Not supported. Not prompted. It is Fundamental. So before you emerge from one more sexual experience singing the blues, here's your pass to climax land. Dumbfounded? Fret not, here's a rundown of sex places that assure incredible climaxes.

Cowgirl

On the off chance that you're physically dynamic and haven't attempted the cowgirl position yet, would you say you are in any event, appreciating it? The individuals who have attempted the cowgirl position, vouch for it. With regards to coming, this is where the cash is at. The cowgirl is the point at which you get on top of your man. Ensure you're kneeling as opposed to crouching to lessen the weight on your thighs. Presently as opposed to bowing forward, recline. Prepare yourself for a stunning O as he rubs you down there. Groan and spread the word!

Switch Cowgirl

What happens when you club cowgirl from the rear? You get the place that will make you shout! Request that your man rests level with his feet somewhat off the bed. As you climb the object of your craving, you can put your hands on his thighs or knees for help. It might appear to be average, however, hang tight for it. Here, his penis will raise a ruckus around town but the champ will be, no award for speculating, YOU! Climb, down, what in tin Theatherze, move around and around! Anything that you do, his joystick will have *all* the delight on the planet. Of course, feet aren't his best element however how about we center around you, will we?

Flatiron

Like from the rear, this position is a much-needed refresher for somebody with a vanilla sexual coexistence. Rests easily on your stomach with knees marginally bowed. Spread your legs and permit him to enter your vagina from behind. Dissimilar to from the rear, this position requires the man to twist towards you. His plonker will dive in deep! This additionally implies you can help yourself. Who is preventing you from making your clit work?

Spooning

What is it that ladies need? Feelings and closeness? Who are we joking with? With regards to sex, what we need the most is the large O. Sexual spooning will, indeed, bring you both. Allow him to be the enormous spoon and enter your vagina from behind. This won't leave a lot of space for development yet it will prod your Sweet spot in the most ideal manner. After you tidy up, you can get back to spooning sans the sex!

Amicability

Feeling overpowered? Get going (and get off) with this piece-of-cake sex position. Place a cushion under your butt to raise your body and charisma. Keep your knees

marginally twisted and spread your legs.
When your man enters you, carry your
knees nearer to your chest and, fold your
legs over him. You both can synchronize the
speed and musicality all the while come.
Once finished, he can fall into your arms as
you kiss and praise the happy climaxes
you've had. Piece of cake, right?

Presently go practice your best ahhs and
oooohs because you will require these
children soon. No more ridin' solo!

www.ingramcontent.com/pod-product-compliance
Lightning Source LLC
Chambersburg PA
CBHW051704250726
48653CB00007B/2841

9798373635479